Chemo Cupcakes and Carpools

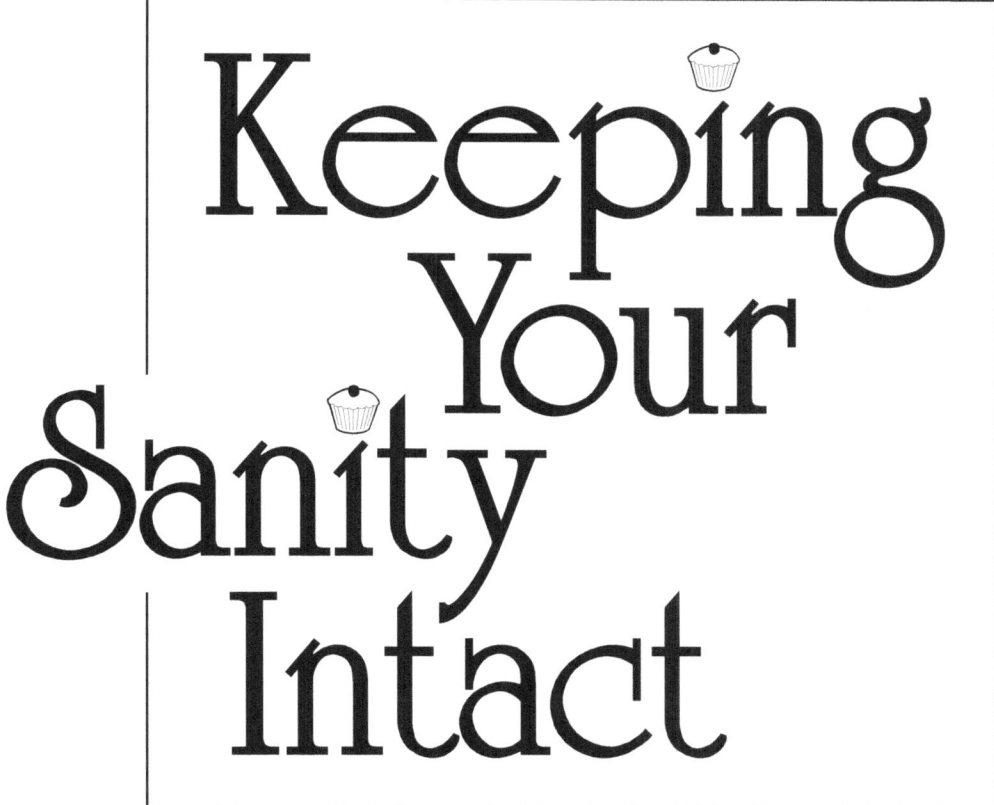

Keeping Your Sanity Intact

ORGANIZER

ANGELIQUE L'AMOUR

Chemo, Cupcakes and Carpool
The Keep Your Sanity Intact
Organizer

ISBN: 978-0-9975444-0-4

Angelique L'Amour
Angelique L'Amour Pitney, Pub
Published by Angelique L'Amour Pitney, Publishing
Los Angeles, CA
Copyright 2016 Angelique L'Amour Pitney
All Rights Reserved

Dedication

To My Fellow Survivors — You are the reason I did this!

Welcome

Welcome to the companion to *Chemo, Cupcakes and Carpools*.
Please write all over this and make sure your family knows about it.
This will help you help them keep it together!

Notes

“ Carpools are a great idea. You can return the favor the next week. Knowing your kids are getting where they need to go frees your brain from worry, and not driving gives you more time to rest and be ready for after school responsibilities. ”
–Angelique L'Amour

Drivers for Kids

Name	Phone/email	Text Y/N

Notes

"There was a spelling bee at school and I decided to go at the last minute. It was two days after chemo and I felt lousy so I asked a neighbor to drive me to school where I sat in the back by the door with a surgical mask on watching my kid compete. I am so glad I didn't miss it because I wasn't up to driving."
–Angelique L'Amour

Drivers for Mom/Dad

Name   Phone/email   Text Y/N

_____

_____

_____

_____

_____

_____

_____

_____

_____

_____

_____

_____

Notes

"You must find the good and the positive in all of it. You must find the humor.
I know it sounds impossible, but the whole situation is impossible, and you are working to fix that.
Try to find a way to look on the bright side or at least don't dwell on the lousy."
–Angelique L'Amour

Gratitude List

Notes

> "Get your hair done. A nice haircut or style will help you feel better before you lose your hair."
> –Angelique L'Amour

Things To Do: Pre-Chemo Appointment List

Appointment	When	Phone/Email

Notes

> *Sometimes it is about eating dessert first. Sometimes you need to treat yourself. One night I was at a party, and everything was too spicy as my mouth sores were active. So I could only eat dessert—honestly, that was the only thing I could eat!*
> *–Angelique L'Amour*

Favorite Foods

_____
_____
_____
_____
_____
_____
_____
_____
_____
_____
_____
_____
_____
_____
_____

Notes

> "Carry water and don't eat without it...Carry protein snacks."
> –Angelique L'Amour

Market List

Notes

> *Start pushing elevator buttons with your knuckles and buy hand sanitizer in bulk for your car, your house, your purse and your kid's backpacks.*
> –Angelique L'Amour

Lunch & Snack

Child	Lunch	Snack

Notes

> *For us it was often easier to just pick up food for dinner. This list will help you keep straight where you like to order from and everyone's favorites.*
> –Angelique L'Amour

Favorite Takeout

Restaurant/Address   Phone   Items

_____
_____
_____
_____
_____
_____
_____
_____
_____
_____
_____
_____
_____
_____

Gratitude Today

Notes

House Numbers

	Name	Phone/email	Text Y/N
Housekeeper			
Dog Walker			
Plumber			
Electrician			
Vet			
Gardner			
Pool			
Neighbor			
Neighbor			
Parents			

Notes

> "You never know when you will need help for your child. It is important to have contact info for teachers, coaches, team parents, etc so you can ask for homework help or a ride to practice."
> –Angelique L'Amour

Kid Numbers

	Name	Phone/email	Text Y/N
Babysitter			
Doctor			
Dentist			
School			
School			
Coach			
Coach			
Teacher			
Teacher			
Grandparents			
Grandparents			

Notes

> *It may be hard at first to accept help, but it is vitally important you accept what is offered and ask for what you really need.*
> –Angelique L'Amour

Kid Activities: What To Take

Kid	Sport/Bag	Food	Day/Time	Where	Team Parent Number

Gratitude Today

Notes

Kid Bath & Hair

Child	Bathtime	Hair

Notes

> " Some young kids have a stuffed friend, blanket, or teddy bear. Tell everyone who helps that this is important and what it is. "
> –Angelique L'Amour

Kid Very Important

Child	Favorite Toy/Book	Can't Live Without

Notes

> *During chemo treatments I started a blog, started a knitting project, found books to read, finished my Christmas shopping.*
> –Angelique L'Amour

Bring to Chemo

- ☐ Snack
- ☐ Beverage(s)
- ☐ Reading material
- ☐ Laptop/Tablet
- ☐ Laptop/Tablet charger
- ☐ Phone
- ☐ Phone charger
- ☐ Glasses
- ☐ Sweater
- ☐ Blanket
- ☐ Pillow

- ☐ _____
- ☐ _____
- ☐ _____
- ☐ _____
- ☐ _____
- ☐ _____
- ☐ _____
- ☐ _____
- ☐ _____
- ☐ _____

Gratitude Today

Notes

What I Felt Like: Chemo Week

	Chemo	Day 2	Day 3	Day 4	Day 5	Day 6	Day 7
Side Effects							
What I Took							
When I Took It							
Did It Work							
Keep or Delete							
When Did I Start To Feel Better							

Notes

> *One of the best pieces of advice I can give you is to write things down. EVERYTHING. Record how you feel after chemo the first time, what medicine you took for side effects, and how you managed the first week. This is your roadmap forward.*
> –Angelique L'Amour

RX That Worked

RX	Chemo	Day 2	Day 3	Day 4	Day 5	Day 6	Day 7
Morning							
Noon							
Night							

Website: angeliquelamour.com

Book: angeliquelamour.com/books/chemo-cupcakes-and-carpools/

 Twitter: @LAmourAngelique

Facebook: www.facebook.com/angeliquelamourauthor

 Instagram: www.instagram.com/angeliquelamourauthor/

Goodreads: Angelique L'Amour

Biography

Angelique L'Amour was born in Los Angeles, California. The daughter of author Louis L'Amour, she grew up in the household of a prolific writer where writing and storytelling were a way of life. In 1988, Angelique created and edited a volume of quotes from her father's works. Published by Bantam Doubleday Dell in 1988, *A Trail of Memories* spent 16 weeks on the *New York Times* bestseller list and was also a *Publisher's Weekly* bestseller for 1988. Angelique has spent the past 20 years as a freelance editor working on academic paper, novels and film projects as well as writing content for two websites. She also created and taught a Creative Writing program for students from 8 to 80 and is contemplating developing that into an online and book course. Future projects include a spiritual self-help book as well as several novels. A wife, mother of two and a breast cancer survivor, time is also spent promoting early detection by teaching, speaking engagements and writing her blog, *My Story Right Now* which can be found through her website: angeliquelamour.com Her current book, *Chemo, Cupcakes and Carpools* is available now wherever books are sold.

Chemo, Cupcakes and Carpools

Keep Your Sanity Intact Organizer

Chemo, Cupcakes and Carpools

Keep Your Sanity Intact Organizer

www.ingramcontent.com/pod-product-compliance
Lightning Source LLC
Chambersburg PA
CBHW060458300426
44113CB00016B/2637